Herbal antibiotics Remedies for Combating Infections.

Rejuvenate your body with healing herbs,overcome any ailments,discover recipes for vibrant health and greater well being.

By

Dr.joe waltern

Many cultures all over the world have used plants as a means of preventing sickness for ages.

The emergence of microorganisms resistant to antibiotics has rekindled interest in herbal medicines today.

This book examines the plants that have been demonstrated to have anti-infective qualities in order to delve into the intriguing science underlying natural antibiotics. In addition, it will explore the background of herbal medicine and offer advice on how to use these all-natural therapies in a secure and efficient manner.

This book provides an extensive examination of herbal antibiotics, whether you're looking for alternate methods of treating common illnesses or you're just interested in the healing properties of plants.

Chapter 1: Overview of Complementary Medicine.

Greetings from the amazing field of herbal medicine! Plants have been used as a natural medicine chest for thousands of years, providing cures for a variety of illnesses.

Herbs have long been used to support health and wellbeing, from licorice root tea to calm lavender to relieve sore throats and anxiety.

We're going to take a journey to discover the essence of herbalism in this chapter. We'll explore its lengthy history, present its possible advantages, and clear up some frequent misunderstandings.

Herbs have been used for medical purposes since the dawn of human civilization.

It has been proven that ancient societies in Mesopotamia,Egypt, China, and India relied on plants for medicinal purposes.

To learn about the medicinal qualities of different plant components, including leaves, roots, flowers, and bark, these early herbalists conducted experiments.

Herbal remedies changed along with knowledge.

Herbs are an integral part of both Traditional Chinese Medicine (TCM) and Ayurveda, an Indian medical system.

 Even the centuries-old humoral hypothesis, which ruled Western medicine, depended on particular herbs to bring the body's fluids back into equilibrium.

The usage of herbal cures decreased as modern medicine emerged in the 19th and 20th centuries.

But because of a growing interest in natural and holistic approaches to health, herbal therapy has seen a comeback in popularity in recent years.

Nature's Bounty: An Examination of the Possible Advantages of Herbs.

Why then are herbs making a comeback? People are rediscovering the potential of plants for the following reasons:

Natural Approach: Herbs provide a drug-free alternative for treating a variety of health issues, and many people prefer natural cures to synthetic drugs.

Focus on the Whole: Rather than only treating symptoms,many people view using herbs as a means of addressing the underlying cause of an illness.

Additionally,they might enhance general wellbeing.

Less negative Effects: Compared to prescription drugs, herbal remedies often have fewer negative effects, though some can still occur.

: A lot of herbs are inexpensive options for healthcare because they are simple to grow at home or get from reliable suppliers.

It's Not Supernatural, But It Has Some Power.

It's critical to approach herbal treatment with reasonable expectations.

Herbs do not treat medical conditions quickly.

But when applied correctly, they can offer a number of advantages:

Supporting the Body's Natural Healing Processes: Herbs have the power to boost immunity, lower inflammation, and facilitate better digestion—all of which help the body heal itself naturally.

Encouraging Overall Wellness: Some herbs have the ability to reduce stress, enhance energy, and increase the quality of sleep, all of which can help one feel better overall.

Offering Effective Relief from Minor Ailments: Herbs can provide effective relief for a range of common problems, from headaches and sore throats to calming coughs and upset stomachs.

Recognizing Your Limitations and Knowing When to Get Professional Assistance

Herbal medicines are an excellent self-care tool, but it's important to be aware of their limitations.

Here are some situations in which getting expert medical advice is crucial:

For severe or long-term medical disorders
Should symptoms worsen or continue even after taking herbs.

Prior to taking herbs combined with prescription drugs if you are expecting or nursing a child.

Recall that using herbal therapy in conjunction with mainstream medicine is a complementary approach.

Before adding herbs to your regimen, always get advice from a licensed healthcare professional, particularly if you have any underlying medical concerns.

You now have a basic understanding of herbal medicine from this chapter.

We'll go deeper into the fascinating realm of natural cures in the upcoming chapters, providing you with the knowledge you need to start your own herbal adventure.

Chapter 2 : Building Your Herb Garden (or Not):Creating a Home Wellness Environment.

Picture yourself going outside your door, picking aromatic mint leaves for a soothing drink, or snipping fresh rosemary for roasted chicken.

Having your own herb garden opens up a world of natural cures at your fingertips, in addition to providing you with wonderful meal complements. But what happens if you're not a green thumb or have a large backyard?

Do not be alarmed, fellow herbalists! This chapter will walk you through the pleasures and things to think about growing your own herb garden, providing advice for individuals with little sunlight or space.

The Enchantment of an In-Growth Herb Garden.

Growing herbs from seed to harvest brings a unique sense of fulfillment.

Observing their development encourages a closer relationship with the medicinal qualities of the plants.

Here are some justifications for thinking about starting a herb garden:

Freshness Is Important: Comparing homegrown herbs to store-bought ones that may have traveled considerable distances, the former are packed with taste and strength.

Constantly Available: Do you need a rapid cure for a stomach ailment or sore throat? A handy natural stress reliever is your own herb garden.

Organic Advantage: You have environmental control and reduce the amount of pesticides and fertilizers you are exposed to.

A Sense of Connection: Planting gardens is a peaceful and fulfilling activity that promotes a sense of accomplishment and a connection with nature.

Making Your Own Herbal Sanctuary:

Let's get your hands filthy now, in the nicest way imaginable!

The following advice will help you create your herb garden:

Location: Pick a sunny area that receives six hours or more of direct sunlight per day. You can grow a herb garden in a container if your patio or balcony receives plenty of sun.

Soil: Fertile, well-drained soil is ideal for herb growth. For the best control over soil quality, think about raised garden beds.

Planting: Learn about each herb's requirements for planting. While some people thrive in warmer climates, others prefer warmer weather. Sort plants that require similar amounts of water together.

Gardening in containers: Lack a yard? Not a problem! For your patio, windowsill, or balcony, go with pots or planters. Select containers that are the right size for the herb and have openings for drainage.

Water your herbs frequently, especially in hot weather, as part of proper herb care. Most herbs want their soil damp, but not wet.

Removing discarded flower petals promotes new development.

Standardized in Sunlight?

Not everyone can get outside in the sun. The following herbs can be grown indoors in bright, indirect light even in shade:

Chamomile: This relaxing plant is excellent for reducing tension and encouraging rest.

Parsley: A multipurpose culinary herb that may help with digestion and breath refreshing.

Mint: Although some varieties spread quickly, others, like peppermint and spearmint, can be successfully cultivated inside in pots under management.

Differential Sourcing:

Maybe you're not very good at gardening, or your living environment prevents you from doing it. The following are sources of fresh herbs:

Farmers markets: Get a colorful assortment of in-season herbs while supporting your neighborhood farmers.

Specialty grocery stores: A greater selection of fresh herbs can be found in specific areas of certain supermarket stores.

Online retailers: A few websites provide pre-packaged fresh herbs or live herb plants that are delivered right to your home.

Regardless of the way you obtain your herbs, this chapter should have ignited your passion for using the power of herbal treatments in your daily life.

Recall that a flourishing herb garden may provide you with great culinary experiences,all-natural wellness.

remedies,and a delightful connection to the restorative force of nature—whether it's growing on a windowsill or in a backyard sanctuary.

Chapter 3: Comprehending Resistance to Antibiotics and Why Herbs Could Be the New Hope.

When you've taken antibiotics for a while, have you ever felt like they didn't really touch your infection?

This situation is becoming more frequent as a result of the growing threat posed by antibiotic resistance.

Once a miraculous treatment, these potent medications are becoming less effective as germs develop resistance to them.

This does not imply that we completely give up on antibiotics.

They remain essential for severe infections.

It does, however, draw attention to the necessity of other strategies.

Herbal treatments are nature's defense against bacterial enemies.

Consider it similar to an arms race.

To survive, bacteria must continually evolve.

Antibiotic abuse and overuse have sped up this process.

Antibiotics are worthless because bacteria build defenses.

Which brings us to now susceptible to infections that were previously treatable with ease.

Thus, what role do herbal therapies play? Unlike conventional antibiotics, a lot of herbs work in many ways.

In addition to killing bacteria, they might also damage their cell walls,interfere with their ability to communicate, or even stop them from adhering to healthy cells.

It is more difficult for bacteria to evolve resistance due to this multifaceted onslaught.

 The body of knowledge regarding herbs' antibacterial qualities is always changing.

Certain plants, such as oregano, thyme, and garlic, have demonstrated potential in combating different types of germs.

Research is also being done on the potential benefits of less well-known herbs, such as goldenseal and echinacea.

It's critical to keep in mind that herbal medicines are not panaceas.

Depending on the particular herb and the kind of infection, they could not be as efficient as antibiotics, and their potency might also change.

But if you include herbs in your wellness regimen, you may be able to:
Boost the defenses of your immune system.

system: Your body's first line of defense against illness is a robust immune system. Some herbs, such as Astragalus and Echinacea, may strengthen your immune system and reduce your susceptibility to illnesses in the first place.

Cut back on the usage of antibiotics: You can prolong the usefulness of antibiotics for more serious cases by taking herbs for minor infections.

Use in conjunction with antibiotics: Sometimes using natural medicines in addition to prescription antibiotics can improve their efficiency.

Here's the important lesson, though: Before using any herbal cure, always get advice from your doctor, especially if you're expecting, nursing, or taking any drugs.

They may offer you advice on the optimal dosage and application as well as assist you decide if a certain herb is good for you.

Herbal treatments provide some hope in the complicated battle against antibiotic resistance.

We can move toward a time when infections are defeated by embracing the power of plants in addition to traditional medicine.

Chapter 4 :Eye-opening Statistics on Alternative Medicine: A Wellness Revolution in the Works.

Ever pop a handful of elderberry candies to stave off a cold, or grab for a warm cup of ginger tea to ease a sore throat?

If so, you're a part of the alternative medicine movement, which is expanding! We'll explore the intriguing world of statistics in this chapter, which shows how people's perspectives on health are changing.

An Increase in Notoriety:

Consider this: A National Center for Health Statistics survey from 2018 revealed that 38% of US individuals used complementary and alternative medicine (CAM) in some capacity.

That is an incredible amount! That means that millions of individuals are looking for complementary natural remedies to traditional medical care.

However, why this spike?

Motives behind the Change:

This tendency is being driven by a number of reasons.

Many individuals are trying to find:

Natural methods: People are becoming more and more interested in natural treatments that are in balance with their bodies.

Empowerment: Individuals desire to be more involved in their own well-being.

Reduced side effects: Some people may look into alternative solutions due to concerns about the possible adverse effects of conventional treatments.

Focus on the whole: Alternative medicine frequently employs a whole approach, treating the underlying cause of a problem as opposed to its symptoms.

What the Data Indicates:

The following startling data, gathered from a variety of sources, gives an overview of this expanding movement:

Herbal Powerhouse: According to a 2020 American Botanical Council research, the US market for herbal supplements reached a staggering $18.9 billion! This demonstrates the enormous interest in plant-based medicine.

Mind-Body Connection: Over 80% of patients receiving conventional cancer treatment also used some sort of complementary and alternative medicine (CAM) therapy, according to a 2021 study published in the Journal of Alternative and Complementary Medicine. This finding highlights the desire for a multimodal approach to health.

The Power of Prevention: According to a 2022 National Institutes of Health (NIH) poll, a sizable percentage of complementary and alternative medicine (CAM) practitioners prioritize preventative care, indicating a proactive attitude to wellness.

Considering the Future:

These figures show a change in the way people view and take care of their health. It's evidence of the increasing interest in natural remedies and a more comprehensive strategy for wellbeing.

We may anticipate that even more people will accept complementary therapy in addition to traditional treatment as long as research on herbal medicines is conducted.

Recall:

Even though these figures are intriguing, it's crucial to speak with a trained healthcare provider before beginning any new herbal medication.

Since each person is different, using natural treatments safely and effectively can only be ensured with expert advice.

We have only begun to explore the fascinating realm of complementary and alternative medicine in this chapter.

In the upcoming chapters, get ready to discover the power of nature's medication!

Chapter 5: Demystifying Antibiotics: An Understanding of the Superpower (and Its Limitations) of Modern Medicine.

Antibiotics: The Cure for Today's Miracle Drugs?

Imagine living in a world where even a minor cut could be fatal.

For a large portion of human history, that was the norm.

Antibiotics brought about a change at the beginning of the 20th century.

These potent drugs transformed medicine by enabling medical professionals to successfully treat a wide range of bacterial infections.

Antibiotics were our go-to tool against these microscopic invaders, treating everything from strep throat to pneumonia.

How Antibiotics Operate: Targeting the Opponent.

Consider bacteria as little factories that are always producing new copies of themselves.

Antibiotics function by interfering with this mechanism in a number of ways.

Some may pierce the bacteria's cell wall, allowing it to leak and eventually perish.

Some people could stop the bacteria from growing, which would halt the infection in its tracks.

When Antibiotics Are Necessary

These drugs are still an essential component of contemporary medicine. Here are a few situations in which antibiotics can actually save lives:

Serious Bacterial Infections: Antibiotics have the potential to save lives in cases of meningitis, pneumonia, and sepsis.

 In order to prevent infections from developing at the surgical site, doctors frequently give antibiotics both before and after surgery.

 The bloodstream may become contaminated with microorganisms as a result of some dental procedures, such as root canals.

Antibiotics assist in keeping this from developing into a dangerous illness.

Antibiotic Resistance's Growing Threat: An Obscuring Shadow.

Antibiotic resistance is a concerning trend that has been brought on by the overuse and abuse of antibiotics.

Because they are intelligent little creatures, bacteria can adapt to survive the very medications meant to destroy them.

As a result, we end up with illnesses that are extremely difficult, if not impossible, to cure.

The Emergence of "Superbugs": "Superbugs," or bacteria resistant to antibiotics, are becoming a greater concern.

These germs are resistant to the potency of our available antibiotics, which has doctors searching for new ways to treat their patients.

Using Antibiotics Sensibly: Keeping Healthy by Fighting Wisely.

How then can you contribute to the solution?

These are important points to keep in mind:

Take Antibiotics Only as Directed: Avoid pressuring your doctor to prescribe antibiotics for a minor illness such as the flu or a cold.

Antibiotics won't help because viruses are the source of them.

Complete the Course: Take the antibiotics as directed for the entire prescribed duration, even if you begin to feel better. If you stop the process early, the germs that survive can return stronger and more resilient.

Consult your physician about available options.

Your doctor may suggest using natural therapies in addition to keeping an eye on your symptoms for some small infections.

Conclusion: Although Effective, Antibiotics Are Not a Miracle Treatment

Although they are an amazing tool in our medical toolbox, antibiotics are not a panacea.

We can efficiently battle illnesses and stop the emergence of antibiotic-resistant superbugs by using them sparingly and investigating complementary methods such as herbal therapies.

The intriguing world of natural antibiotics—those plant warriors hiding in your kitchen or garden—will be explored in the upcoming chapter.

Chapter 6: Using Herbs to Fight Infection: Nature's Arsenal.

People have used plants as medicine for generations.

Even with the wonders of contemporary medicine at our fingertips,many people still choose herbal therapies.

The possibility that some herbs could function as natural antibiotics is among the strongest arguments in favor of this ongoing interest.

Let's clear the air before you start thinking of these as some sort of miraculous substitute for antibiotics that your doctor has given.

As currently understood, true antibiotics are potent drugs that specifically target certain germs.

They are an essential weapon against dangerous illnesses.

However, antibiotic resistance is a developing issue as a result of the misuse of conventional antibiotics.

Since bacteria are always changing, certain strains have evolved to be resistant to the effects of antibiotics.

This increases the difficulty of treating infections.

This is where herbs with possible antibacterial qualities, or natural antibiotics more precisely, come into play.

Consider them to be nature's first defense. While there may not be a single herb that works for everyone, several can strengthen your immune system and assist your body fight off infections by themselves.

Furthermore, some herbs may have qualities that directly prevent some bacterial strains from growing.

A glimpse inside the medicinal cupboard of nature:

Garlic: A well-known immune system stimulant, garlic is a pungent powerhouse. Research indicates that it might possess antimicrobial qualities against many types of bacteria, such as Staphylococcus aureus and E. Coli.

Ginger: This adaptable root helps with more than simply sickness.

According to research, ginger may be useful in treating some foodborne infections due to its antibacterial properties.

Honey: For centuries, people have valued the therapeutic qualities of nature's golden nectar.

Honey has special antibacterial qualities that can aid in the topical treatment of infections, such as small wounds.

Echinacea: For generations, people have utilized this well-known herb to strengthen their immune systems. Some evidence suggests it may lessen the duration of colds and flu, but more research is needed to determine how effective it is against specific diseases.

Goldenseal: This herb native to North America has long been used as a remedy for a number of ailments.

Further research is necessary to determine its efficiency,but some studies indicate that it may have antibacterial capabilities against particular strains of bacteria.

It's important to keep in mind that herbal medicines should never be used in place of medical advice from a professional.

See your doctor as soon as possible if you think you may have a dangerous infection.

Consider natural antibiotics as partners in maintaining your general health.

 It may be possible to support your body's natural defenses and ward against infections by including these herbs in your diet or utilizing them in the right preparations.

Recall: To make sure herbal treatments are safe and suitable for you, seek the advice of a licensed herbalist or healthcare provider before experimenting with them.

Chapter 7: Nature's Little Green Medicine Cabinet: The Top 45 Wonder Herbs.

Have you ever searched in your kitchen cupboards for a herbal cure?

Perhaps a warm salt water gargle for a sore throat or some of granny's comforting ginger tea for an unsettled stomach?

If so, you've already taken a tentative step into the fascinating realm of herbal treatments!

This chapter serves as your personal guide to 45 amazing wonder plants found in nature.

We'll look at their conventional usage as well as prospective advantages,but keep in mind that this material should never be used in place of expert medical advice.

Before beginning any new herbal therapy, always get medical advice, especially if you have any underlying medical concerns or are currently taking prescription.

A preview of some of the incredible herbs we'll be revealing: For Relieved Digestive System:

Peppermint: This cooling plant helps relieve indigestion, relieve heartburn, and settle an upset stomach.

Ginger: A potent antidote to nausea, ginger also helps promote regular digestion and lessen bloating.

Chamomile: This herb is useful not only for relaxation but also for reducing pain and cramping in the stomach.
Regarding Respiratory Assistance:

Echinacea: When taken as soon as symptoms appear, this well-known plant may help reduce how long colds and the flu last.

Elderberry: Packed with antioxidants, elderberries can help with colds, congestion, and coughing.

Thyme: This aromatic herb contains expectorant qualities that help loosen mucus and ease coughing.

To Unwind and Fall asleep:

Lavender: Lavender, with its relaxing scent, is known to reduce anxiety and encourage sound sleep.

Valerian Root: For centuries, people have used this plant to help them relax and get better sleep.

Another herb that has a relaxing effect is passionflower, which may also help alleviate anxiety and improve sleep.
Regarding General Well-Being:

Garlic: Packed with health benefits, garlic may help maintain heart health and a strong immune system.

Turmeric: Rich in anti-inflammatory qualities, this golden spice may improve joint health and general wellbeing.

Nettle Leaf: Iron-rich and high in vitamins and minerals, nettle leaf also helps maintain normal blood pressure.
This is only a small sampling of the amazing array of miraculous plants that are out there.

As we go farther, we'll examine each plant in greater detail and provide details about:
Common Names: We've included the most well-known names for herbs that you may be familiar with.

Possible Advantages: Drawing from the literature, we will talk about the historical applications and possible health advantages of each herb.

Recall that your herbal journey is only getting started.

You may naturally enhance your general well-being and tap into the power of nature's medical cabinet with a little research and direction.

Now pick up your herbal teacup, open this page, and let's go on this adventure!

Chapter 8: Unknown Herbal Cure Recipes: Your Kitchen as Nature's Pharmacy.

Imagine waking up with a scratchy throat—a surefire indicator that a cold is about to set in.

Alternatively, perhaps you overate at supper and are now experiencing stomach pains.

Give your own kitchen some thought before reaching for any over-the-counter drugs!

This chapter explores the world of lesser-known herbal cure remedies, turning everyday items from your cupboard into health-promoting natural friends.

Let's take a tour through a few easy yet powerful mixtures:

1. Tea for Soothing Sore Throat:

Do you have that itchy, scratchy feeling? This drink made of herbs could be your savior.

In a cup of boiling water, steep one tablespoon of dried sage leaves and one teaspoon of dried marshmallow root.

for ten minutes. Pour through a strainer, squeeze in some honey (for a calming sweetness), and drink this hot tea multiple times over the day. While marshmallow root covers the throat to reduce inflammation, sage has inherent antibacterial qualities.

2. Distressed Stomach Remedy:

Do you feel sick to your stomach? Superhero in the herbal world, ginger, steps in to save the day.

All you have to do is grate a piece of fresh ginger like the size of your thumb into a cup of boiling water.

After five minutes of steeping, drain and, if preferred, squeeze in a few drops of lemon juice.

You can reduce nausea and relax your stomach with this easy ginger tea.

3. The Booster for Immunity:

Are you exhausted? Elderberry and echinacea,two herbs with potential immune-boosting qualities, combine their deliciousness in this strong blend.

 A teaspoon of dried echinacea root and a handful of dried elderberries should be simmered in two cups of water for fifteen minutes in a pot.

Strain the mixture, drizzle with honey, and sip this warm beverage every day—especially in the winter when colds and flu are on the rise.

4. Soothing Bath with Lavender:

Are you under stress? Make your bathtub a relaxing sanctuary.

Gather some dried lavender flowers and tie them into a sachet using cheesecloth.

Pour the lavender sachet into a warm bath and allow the relaxing scent to do its job.

With addition to its well-known calming effects, lavender's aroma can aid with sensations of calmness and serenity.

5. Homemade Calendula Cream:

You have a small cut or scrape? The daisy-like flower calendula may have skin-soothing qualities.

Calendula flowers are infused into olive oil using a gentle heat process for several weeks to form a salve (see "infused oil" for further details).

To make a salve, strain the oil and combine it with beeswax.

To aid in healing, apply a thin layer to the injured region.

Keep in mind that these recipes are only the beginning!

Try experimenting with different flavors and herbs to see which ones suit you the best.

Important Information: If you are pregnant, nursing, or on any drugs, talk to your doctor before using any herbal remedies.

You can use these simple recipes and a little ingenuity to use nature's healing powers to treat minor illnesses and enhance general health.

Thus, keep in mind that your kitchen may have the secret to natural healing the next time you're feeling under the weather!

Chapter 9: Using Nature's Little Warriors to Naturally Fight Common Ailments.

Do you feel unwell? You may find yourself reaching for the pharmaceutical cabinet if you have a persistent cough or a sore throat that sounds like sandpaper.

But before you reach for that bottle of cherry-flavored or bright pink beverage, remember the strength of nature's own remedy: herbs!

Numerous herbs have remarkable qualities that can boost your body's natural healing process and help reduce discomfort.

Imagine them as tiny green (or occasionally colorful) warriors collaborating with your immune system to fend off intruders.

Here, we'll look at a few typical illnesses and the herbal heroes that can help you:

Colds & Flu: Do you feel blocked up and achy? This traditional pair can be addressed with a multifaceted herbal strategy.

Echinacea: If taken as soon as symptoms appear, this well-known plant may help lessen the duration and intensity of a cold.

Elderberry: Packed with antioxidants, elderberry syrup has the potential to both prevent and treat influenza symptoms, such as fever and congestion.

Ginger: Not only does this miracle reduce nausea, but it also relieves sore throats and coughs. For a soothing pick-me-up, sip some ginger tea with a touch of lemon and honey.

Peppermint: Do you have congestion? Tea with peppermint leaves can help reduce mucus and the stuffy feeling. Take a breath in the steam rising from a cup for added cleansing.

Digestive Discomfort: Do you feel swollen, bloated, or do you have cramping in your stomach? Remain optimistic! The following herbal companions can help you restore your digestive system:

Peppermint: This adaptable plant eases the tension in your digestive system's muscles.

relieving dyspepsia and reducing cramping.

Ginger: Ginger is an incredible remedy for nausea and vomiting. Savor it with chews,tea, or even mixed into a calming broth.

Chamomile: This soothing plant can help reduce anxiety and upset stomach, which are frequently linked to digestive problems.

Fennel Seed: Drinking tea made from fennel seeds might help reduce gas and bloating and make you feel lighter.

Sore Throat: It can be rather unpleasant to have that itchy, uncomfortable feeling in your throat. The following plants can help ease the discomfort:

Licorice Root: This herb with a pleasant taste and anti-inflammatory qualities might help soothe sore throats. However, be advised that licorice root may interact with certain drugs, so consult your physician before taking it.

Slippery Elm: This herb relieves dryness and irritation in the throat by coating it with a calming mucilage. Drink some slippery elm tea to help you relax.

Sage: To reduce swelling and soreness in the throat, gargle with sage tea.

Recall:

Even though these herbs have certain benefits, it's crucial to pay attention to your health.

Always seek medical advice if symptoms worsen or persist.

Herbal medicines' efficacy varies from person to person.

What is extremely effective for one individual may not have the same impact on another.

Try several things to see what suits you the best!

Before using herbs,it is important to see a doctor, especially if you are on medication, are pregnant, or are nursing a baby.

By adding these herbal warriors to your regimen,you can give your body the tools it needs to naturally combat common illnesses and recover more quickly.

Keep in mind that nature has gifted us with an amazing collection of medicinal plants; therefore,the next time you're feeling under the weather, think about trying these plant-powered remedies!

Chapter 10: Nature's Gifts with Gently Guidance: An Understanding of Herb Safety and Interactions.

Greetings from the amazing world of herbal treatments once again!

We've looked into the intriguing past of these plant allies, learned how to grow or obtain them, and even investigated the effectiveness of organic antibiotics.

Let's first discuss safety and interactions before you go crazy and stock your herb cupboard.

Consider herbs as strong allies. They provide amazing assistance,but like any friend, they may not always get along with everyone in your life, especially prescription drugs.

Although herbs are generally safe when used as directed, it is important to be aware of potential interactions and negative effects.

Not Every Herb Is Made Equal
First of all, keep in mind that the potency of herbs varies.

Strong St John's Wort tincture for mood support may be quite different from a mild chamomile tea for relaxation.

Always begin with a little dose and raise it gradually to see how your body reacts.

Herbal-Medicine Interactions: A Fine Dance.

This is where things can become a little more complex.

Certain herbs may interact with prescription drugs that you may be taking. Grapefruit juice, for instance,may conflict with some statins that are prescribed to lower cholesterol.

Popular cold-remedy herb echinacea may interact with blood thinners.

The golden rule is this: Always talk to your doctor or other healthcare provider about any herbal remedies you are thinking about using.

Regarding possible interactions between your drugs and medical problems, they can provide you with advice.

Typical Side Effects: What to Anticipate
Similar to any medication, there may be adverse effects from herbs.

Depending on the herb, dosage, and individual sensitivity, they can be moderate to severe.

The following are some typical adverse effects to be aware of:

Uneasy stomach: Certain herbs may result in queasiness, vomiting, or diarrhea.
Headaches: When used in larger dosages, several plants may cause headaches.
Reactions due to allergies: Although rare, certain plants may cause allergic reactions in certain persons. If you have a known allergy to plants, proceed with caution.

Interactions between drugs: This is a very important issue, as was previously stated!

Who Is It Safe to Use Certain Herbs?
Although there are many advantages to using herbs, the following groups may need to take particular care:

Women who are pregnant or nursing: Some herbs may not be safe to use during these times.

Whenever possible, get medical advice before using any herbs during this time.

Children: It's advisable to avoid providing strong herbs to children without first contacting a pediatrician because their bodies are still developing.

Individuals suffering from severe medical conditions: See your doctor about any herbal treatments you may be taking if you have a chronic condition or are receiving treatment to ensure safety.

Prioritizing Safety Your Herbal Adventure Begins Here.

Knowing possible interactions and adverse effects will help you confidently traverse the world of herbs.

Here are some more pointers for using herbs safely:

Purchase from reliable vendors: Select premium, organic herbs from reputable retailers or herbalists.

Pay close attention to the labels: Observe the dosing guidelines and cautions.

Begin slowly and at a low volume: Start with a little dosage and raise it gradually as necessary.

Pay attention to your body. Stop using the product and speak with your doctor if you encounter any unfavorable side effects.

Maintain a record: Keep a record of the herbs you take and give it to your physician.

Recall that information is power! Through thorough investigation and candid dialogue with your medical professional, you may use the potential of herbs while guaranteeing a secure and fulfilling herbal journey.

Now, confidently venture forth and discover this fascinating realm of natural wellbeing!

Chapter 11: A Handbook for Aspiring Herbalists on the Responsible Harvesting, Storing, and Sourcing of Herbs.

Greetings from the amazing world of herbal treatments once again! It's likely that by this point you've come upon a veritable gold mine of herbs that can help relieve your pain, strengthen your immune system, and promote your general health.

But let's talk about how to handle these plant partners responsibly before you go all in making a powerful concoction.

You may confidently harvest, store, and source your herbs with the help of this chapter.

From Herb Garden to Jar: Gathering Herbs the Correct Way.

Picture cutting fresh rosemary from your herb garden and inhaling its heady scent. It's a lovely picture, and gathering your own herbs makes you feel more.

Connected to the environment. These are a few pointers for an effective harvest:
Recognize When to Harvest: Herbs have varying peak potencies, which should be noted.

Find out when is the best time to harvest each herb.

In general, it is ideal to harvest flowers right before they blossom, whereas leaves are best taken early in the morning, once the dew has evaporated.

Show Plant Respect: Avoid becoming avaricious! To ensure the plant continues to develop, take only what you need, leaving at least one-third of the plant left.

It's acceptable to harvest the top third of the stems on taller plants.

Sharp is secure: Harvest your herbs with sterile, sharp instruments, such as pruning shears.

This reduces plant damage and encourages clean cutting.

Maintaining the Potency: Preserving Your Herbs for Future Use.

After gathering your priceless herbs, it's time to make sure they stay potent so you can use them later. Here are a few essential storage techniques:

Drying: This is the most widely used technique.

Wash your herbs gently, pat them dry, and hang them in a cool, dark, well-ventilated room.

Bundles can be tied with string or placed on drying racks.

After they are dry, store them in cool, dark places in airtight containers.

Freezing: Freezing is a good way to preserve certain herbs, such as basil and mint.

After washing and finely chopping, place them in a single layer on a baking sheet and place them in the freezer.

After they're frozen firm, move them to airtight jars.

Oils Infused: Hold the Essence of Your fave oilseed herbs.

Your preferred herb, either fresh or dried, should be added to a sterilized jar and completely covered with premium olive oil.

For many weeks, store the jar in a cold, dark area with occasional shaking.

Tightly seal the jar.

How to Select Herbs Sensibly: Where to Look for Your Botanical Allies.

Not everyone has the time or room to grow herbs.

Fortunately, there are additional options for obtaining premium herbs.

Here are a few choices:

Regional farmers markets Herbs grown organically or using sustainable resources are a specialty of many farms.

This keeps your herbs fresh and helps you support small businesses in your community.

Reputable Herbal Stores: Seek out establishments that have an emphasis on ethical sourcing methods and have staff members who are equipped to address your inquiries.

Internet-based retailers: Online shopping might be easy, but proceed with caution. Select trustworthy suppliers with good ratings and open sourcing policies.

A Word of Caution: Unless you can positively identify them, always stay away from wild-grown herbs.

It's advisable to stick to trustworthy suppliers because some plants have dangerous lookalikes.

You and Your Herbs for Safe and Responsible Herbalism.

Recall that adverse effects are possible with even natural therapies.

Here are a few last things to think about:

: Any herbal supplementation should always be discussed with your doctor, especially if you are also taking medicine.

Start modest, Go Slow: When taking new herbs in particular, start with a modest dosage and see how your body responds before gradually increasing.

Quality Is Important Whenever possible, use herbs that are sourced sustainably or organically.

As a result, there is a lower chance of being exposed to toxins and pesticides.

You can learn to use the power of nature as a responsible herbalist who respects the environment and looks out for your own health by adopting these techniques. With this knowledge at your disposal, venture out and discover the fascinating realm of herbal treatments!

Conclusion

Natural medicines have an irresistible charm.

However, don't allow herbal remedies to be a false hope in cases of severe infections.

Investigate natural remedies in addition to conventional medication, not in instead of it, and follow your doctor's advice.

Recall that having the appropriate treatment plan is essential to protecting your health, which is a priceless gift.

www.ingramcontent.com/pod-product-compliance
Lightning Source LLC
Chambersburg PA
CBHW081539250726
48659CB00009B/3000